GUIDE TO HEART DISEASE PREVENTION

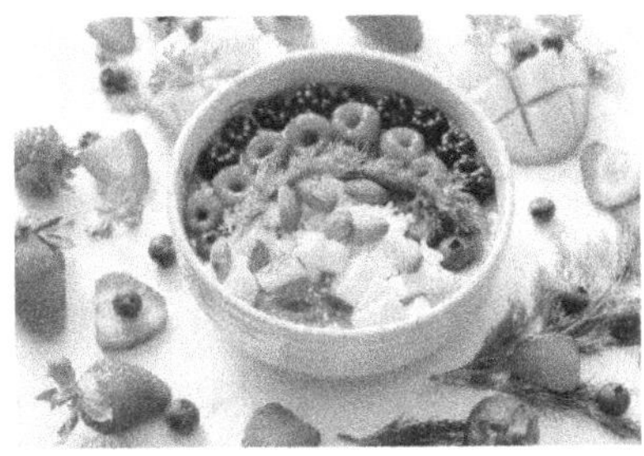

Over 100 easy Mediterranean diet recipes to achieve healthier health.

BY
AUDREY PARKER

Table of contents

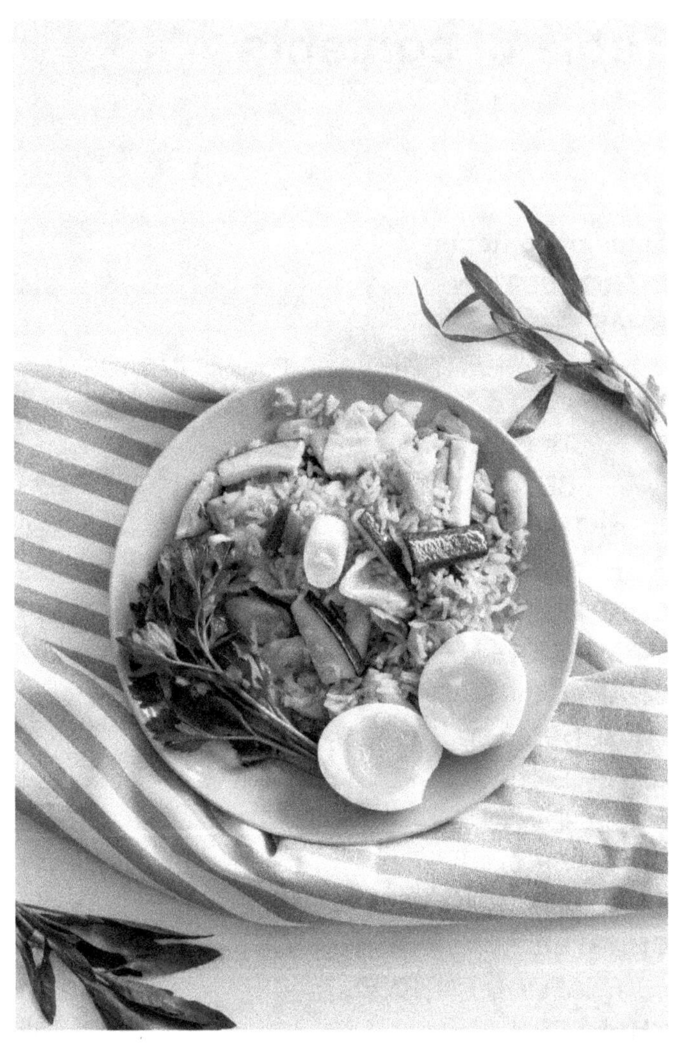

INTRODUCTION

Welcome to the profound exploration of heart health—an indispensable journey through the intricacies of cardiovascular well-being. The heart, that relentless and vital organ, serves as the rhythmic conductor orchestrating the symphony of life within us. As we navigate the complex landscape of modern living, it becomes imperative to understand the dynamics of heart disease, an ailment that looms ominously in the shadows of our fast-paced existence.

Heart disease, a collective term for various conditions affecting the heart and blood vessels, stands as a formidable adversary in the realm of health. From coronary artery disease to heart failure, its manifestations vary, yet they all share a common thread—a threat to the ceaseless rhythm of our life force. This silent assailant often creeps stealthily, exhibiting minimal symptoms until it reaches a critical juncture, underscoring the importance of proactive measures in its prevention.

The stakes are high, and the significance of cultivating a healthy heart cannot be overstated. A robust cardiovascular system not only fuels the body with oxygen and nutrients but also acts as the linchpin in maintaining overall well-being. A heart in peak condition pulsates with vitality, fostering resilience against the trials of time and external stressors.

Embracing a lifestyle that champions heart health is akin to investing in a sustainable future for our most vital organ. It entails a holistic approach that extends beyond fleeting fads, emphasizing the enduring impact of dietary choices, physical activity, stress management, and overall self-care. The quest for a healthy heart is not merely a matter of extending longevity but enhancing the quality of life—a pursuit that pays dividends in energy, resilience, and the sheer joy of living.

In this enlightening journey, we will unravel the multifaceted aspects of heart disease prevention, empowering you with knowledge and actionable insights. From dietary patterns that resonate with the Mediterranean allure to the significance of regular exercise, stress reduction techniques, and the vigilance required in understanding risk factors, this exploration is a compass guiding you toward the shores of cardiovascular well-being.

So, embark on this odyssey with an open heart—both metaphorically and literally—as we unravel the secrets, dispel the myths, and celebrate the magnificence of a healthy heart. The beats of life are counting on it, and the symphony awaits its conductor—YOU.

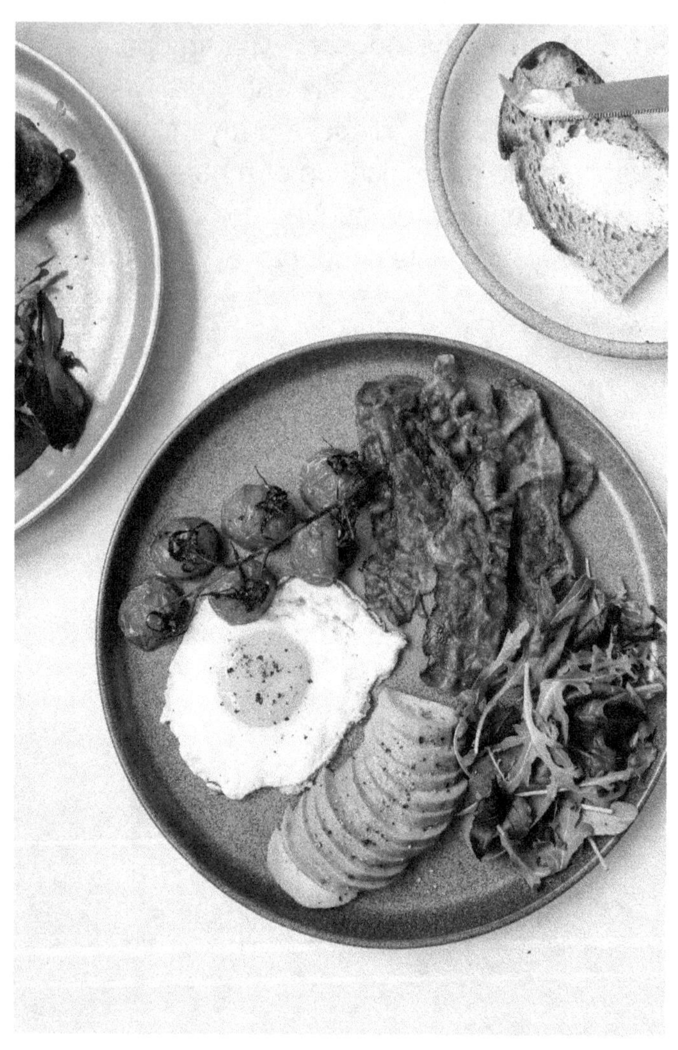

CHAPTER 1

AVOID HEART DISEASE BY EATING RIGHT

Preventing heart disease through food is not just a dietary choice; it's a powerful strategy to fortify your cardiovascular health. Adopting a heart-healthy diet involves making mindful selections that support your heart's well-being.

Studies have shown that the best plan for following a heart-healthy way of eating is the Mediterranean diet. Embrace the following principles to create a nourishing and protective culinary foundation:

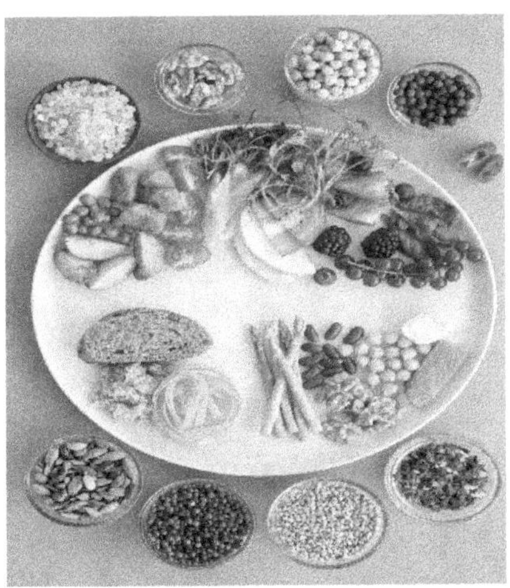

Mediterranean Marvel:

Channel the Mediterranean diet, rich in fruits, vegetables, whole grains, and healthy fats like olive oil. This dietary pattern has been lauded for its ability to reduce the risk of heart disease by promoting good cholesterol levels and lowering blood pressure.

Omega-3 Rich Fare:

Prioritize foods abundant in omega-3 fatty acids, such as fatty fish (salmon, mackerel, and sardines), flaxseeds, chia seeds, and walnuts. These fats have been shown to support heart health by reducing inflammation and enhancing blood vessel function.

Colorful Bounty:

Embrace a spectrum of colorful fruits and vegetables. They are not only rich in vitamins and minerals but also packed with antioxidants that combat oxidative stress, a contributor to heart disease.

Whole Grains Galore:

Choose whole grains such as oats, quinoa, and brown rice. These grains provide essential fiber, which aids in lowering cholesterol levels and maintaining a healthy weight.

Lean Protein Choices:

Choose lean protein sources like poultry, fish, legumes, and tofu. Limit red meat consumption and opt for healthier protein alternatives to reduce saturated fat intake.

Mindful Portion Control:

To maintain a healthy weight, pay attention to portion sizes. Overeating, even of nutritious foods, can contribute to obesity, a significant risk factor for heart disease.

Ditch the Trans Fats:

Minimize or eliminate trans fats found in many processed and fried foods. These fats can raise bad cholesterol levels (LDL) and increase the risk of coronary artery disease.

Limit Added Sugars and Salt:

Reduce your intake of added sugars and sodium. Excessive salt can elevate blood pressure, while too much sugar contributes to weight gain and metabolic issues, both detrimental to heart health.

Hydration Matters:

Stay well-hydrated with water. Adequate hydration supports overall health and can aid in weight management, indirectly benefiting heart health.

Spice it Up:

Experiment with heart-friendly herbs and spices like garlic, turmeric, and cinnamon. These not only enhance flavor but also offer potential cardiovascular benefits.

Common Risk Factors

There are common risk factors for heart disease you should know about and they include the following:

- Poor diet
- Physical inactivity
- Smoking and Tobacco Use
- Excessive Alcohol Consumption
- Obesity
- High Blood Pressure(Hypertension)
- High Cholesterol
- Diabetes
- Sleep deprivation
- Stress

Most Common Types Of Heart Diseases In The World Today

A variety of disorders affecting the heart and blood vessels are included in the category of heart disease. These are a few of the most typical kinds:

Coronary Artery Disease (CAD):

The most common kind of heart disease is this one. CAD occurs when the blood vessels (coronary arteries) that supply blood to the heart muscle become narrowed or blocked by cholesterol and other deposits, restricting blood flow.

Heart Failure:

Heart failure doesn't mean the heart has stopped beating, but rather that it's not pumping blood as effectively as it should. It can result from conditions like CAD, high blood pressure, or previous heart attacks.

Arrhythmias:

Arrhythmias are irregular heartbeats. They can manifest as tachycardia (too fast), bradycardia (too slow), or irregular rhythms. While some are harmless, others can be life-threatening.

Valve Disorders:

Problems with the heart valves can impede blood flow. Conditions include stenosis

(narrowing) or regurgitation (leakage), often
caused by aging or infections.

Cardiomyopathy:

This condition involves the enlargement or
thickening of the heart muscle, making it
harder for the heart to pump blood. It can be
genetic or result from other conditions.

Peripheral Artery Disease (PAD):

PAD occurs when there's a buildup of plaque in
the arteries that supply blood to the limbs,
often leading to reduced blood flow to the legs
and feet.

Myocardial Infarction (Heart Attack):

When a blood clot, usually, blocks blood flow to
a portion of the heart muscle, the result is a
heart attack. It may permanently harm the
heart muscle.

Hypertrophic Cardiomyopathy:

This is a genetic condition where the heart muscle thickens, making it harder for the heart to pump blood. It's a common cause of sudden cardiac arrest in young people.

Rheumatic Heart Disease:

Rheumatic fever, usually resulting from inadequately treated strep throat, can lead to rheumatic heart disease. It causes damage to the heart valves.

Congenital Heart Defects:

These are structural heart problems present at birth. They may impact the blood vessels, valves, or chambers of the heart.

Understanding the specific type of heart disease is crucial for appropriate management and treatment. Prevention strategies often involve lifestyle changes, medication, and, in some cases, surgical interventions. Regular medical check-ups and consultations with healthcare professionals are essential for early detection and effective management of heart-related conditions.

BEYOND THE PLATE

"Beyond the plate" signifies the recognition that cultivating heart health extends far beyond mere dietary choices. It encompasses a holistic approach that considers various aspects of lifestyle and well-being. Here are key dimensions that go beyond the plate in promoting heart health:

Physical Activity:

Regular exercise is a cornerstone of heart health. Physical activity strengthens the heart muscle, improves circulation, and helps manage weight, blood pressure, and cholesterol levels.

Stress Management:

Chronic stress can contribute to heart disease. Practices like meditation, mindfulness, and relaxation techniques are essential for managing stress and promoting overall well-being.

Adequate Sleep:

Quality sleep is crucial for heart health. Lack of sleep has been linked to conditions such as obesity, high blood pressure, and diabetes, all of which contribute to heart disease.

Tobacco Cessation:

Quitting smoking and avoiding tobacco products is one of the most impactful ways to reduce the risk of heart disease. Smoking causes vascular damage and raises the risk of atherosclerosis.

Moderation in Alcohol Consumption:

While moderate alcohol consumption may have some cardiovascular benefits, excessive drinking can contribute to high blood pressure, heart failure, and other heart-related issues.

Regular Health Check-ups:

Periodic health check-ups help monitor key indicators of heart health, such as blood pressure, cholesterol levels, and blood sugar levels. Early detection allows for timely intervention.

Weight Management:

Maintaining a healthy weight reduces the strain on the heart and lowers the risk of conditions like hypertension and diabetes, which are significant contributors to heart disease.

Hydration:

Staying adequately hydrated supports overall health and helps the heart pump blood more efficiently. Water is essential for various bodily functions, including those related to the cardiovascular system.

Social Connections:

Building and maintaining meaningful social connections can contribute to emotional well-being. Strong social ties have been associated with a lower risk of heart disease.

Regular Health Screenings:

Beyond routine check-ups, specific health screenings, such as cholesterol tests, blood pressure checks, and diabetes screenings, are crucial for early detection and prevention.

Avoiding Illicit Drug Use:

Substance abuse, including the use of illicit drugs, can have detrimental effects on heart health. Avoiding such substances is essential for maintaining cardiovascular well-being.

Embracing these lifestyle factors in addition to a heart-healthy diet forms a comprehensive strategy for preventing heart disease and promoting overall cardiovascular wellness. The interplay of these elements fosters a balanced and sustainable approach to living that goes beyond the confines of the plate.

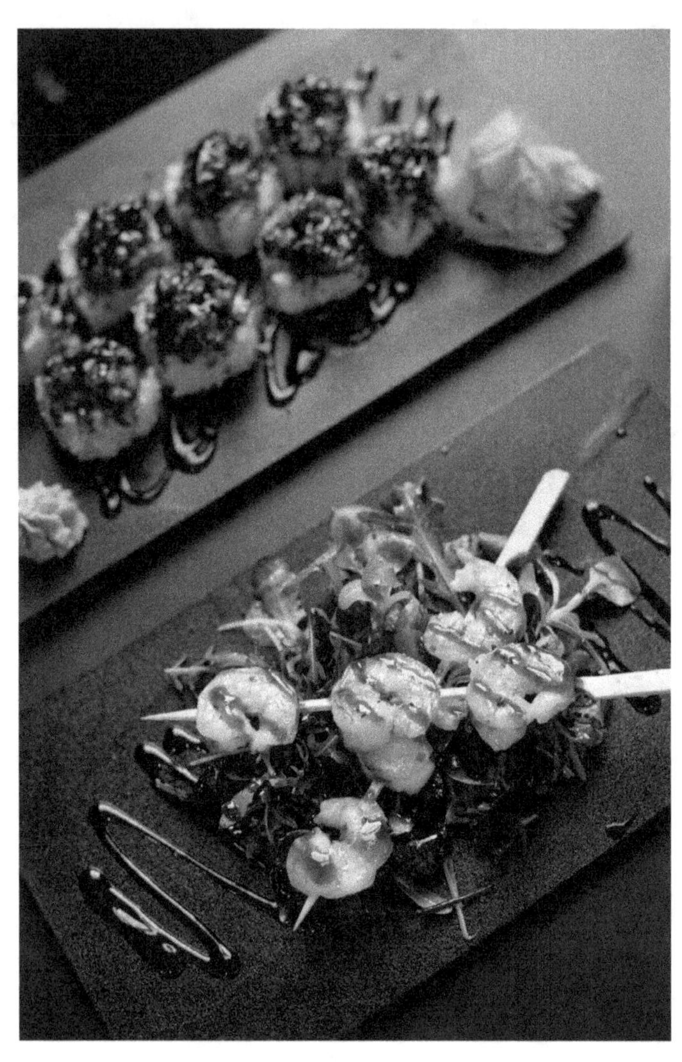

CHAPTER 2

Heart-Healthy Breakfasts:

1. **Greek Yogurt Parfait:**
   - 1 cup of Greek yogurt
   - Mixed berries (blueberries, strawberries)
   - 1 tablespoon of chia seeds
   - A drizzle of honey
   - Granola for crunch
2. **Vegetable Omelet:**
   - 2 eggs (whisked)
   - Spinach, tomatoes, and bell peppers (chopped)
   - Feta cheese (optional)
   - Whole-grain toast on the side
3. **Overnight Chia Seed Pudding:**
   - 3 tablespoons chia seeds
   - 1 cup almond milk
   - Sliced mango and kiwi for topping
   - Almonds or walnuts for added crunch
4. **Avocado Toast:**
   - Whole-grain toast
   - Mashed avocado
   - Sliced tomatoes

- Sprinkle of black pepper and a dash of olive oil

5. **Quinoa Breakfast Bowl:**
   - Cooked quinoa
   - Mixed with almond milk
   - Topped with sliced bananas, berries, and a dollop of Greek yogurt

Heart-Friendly Beverages:

1. **Berry Blast Smoothie:**
   - Ingredients: Mixed berries, spinach, Greek yogurt, and a splash of coconut water.
   - Instructions: Blend ingredients until smooth for a nutrient-packed, refreshing smoothie.
2. **Herbal Tea Infusion:**
   - Ingredients: Hibiscus or chamomile tea bag, hot water, and a slice of lemon.
   - Instructions: Steep the tea bag, add a slice of lemon, and enjoy a calming herbal infusion.

3. **Iced Green Tea with Citrus:**
   - Ingredients: Green tea, ice cubes, lemon slices, and mint leaves.
   - Instructions: Brew green tea, let it cool, add ice cubes, and garnish with lemon slices and mint leaves.
4. **Golden Milk Latte:**
   - Ingredients: Turmeric, almond milk, honey, and a pinch of black pepper.
   - Instructions: Warm almond milk with turmeric, honey, and black pepper for a comforting, anti-inflammatory beverage.
5. **Watermelon Mint Cooler:**
   - Ingredients: Fresh watermelon chunks, mint leaves, and sparkling water.
   - Instructions: Muddle mint leaves, mix with watermelon, and top with sparkling water for a hydrating and refreshing drink.

These examples provide a variety of nutrient-rich options for a heart-healthy start to your day. Feel free to customize them based on your preferences and dietary needs.

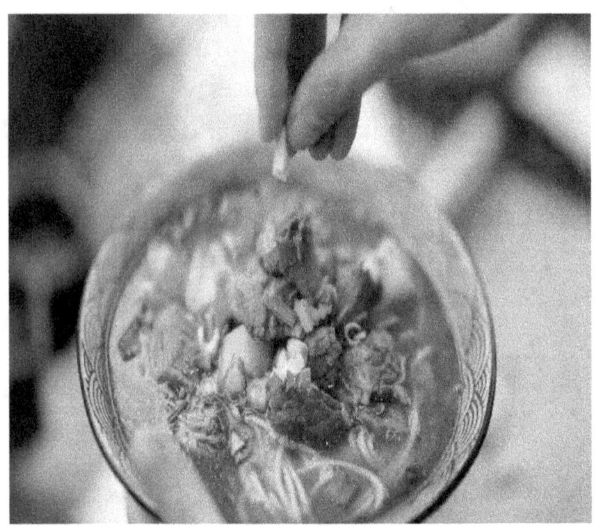

CHAPTER 3

MEZZE DISHES

Mezze" refers to a selection of small dishes served as appetizers in parts of the Middle East, Mediterranean, and some Balkan countries. It's a delightful way to experience a variety of flavors and textures. Here are a few classic mezze dishes you might enjoy:

Hummus:

- A smooth blend of chickpeas, tahini, lemon juice, and garlic, drizzled with olive oil. Perfect for dipping with pita bread or veggies.

Baba Ganoush:

- Smoky eggplant dip made with roasted eggplant, tahini, garlic, lemon juice, and olive oil.

Tzatziki:

- A Greek yogurt-based dip with cucumber, garlic, dill, and olive oil. Refreshing and great with grilled meats or as a dip.

Tabbouleh:

- A parsley salad with tomatoes, mint, onion, and soaked bulgur, dressed with olive oil and lemon juice.

Falafel:

- Deep-fried balls made from ground chickpeas or fava beans, usually served with tahini sauce.

Dolma:

- ○ Grape leaves stuffed with a mixture of rice, pine nuts, and herbs. Sometimes stuffed with minced meat.

Muhammara:

- ○ A Syrian dip made with red peppers, walnuts, garlic, and olive oil, blended to a smooth consistency.

Labneh:

- ○ Strained yogurt with a thick, creamy texture. Often served with a drizzle of olive oil and herbs.

Olives and Feta:

- A simple combination of marinated olives and feta cheese, sometimes with herbs or citrus zest.

Sambousek:

- Small savory pastries filled with ingredients like spiced meat, cheese, or spinach.

Grilled Halloumi:

- Grilled slices of halloumi cheese, often served with a squeeze of lemon.

Moutabal:

- Similar to baba ganoush, moutabal is an eggplant dip but may include yogurt, tahini, or garlic for added creaminess and flavor.

Kibbeh:

- Ground meat (often lamb or beef) mixed with bulgur, onions, and spices. It can be shaped into patties or balls and either baked or fried.

Mezze dishes are meant to be shared, creating a communal and convivial dining experience. They offer a diverse array of flavors and textures, making them a delightful part of Mediterranean and Middle Eastern culinary traditions.

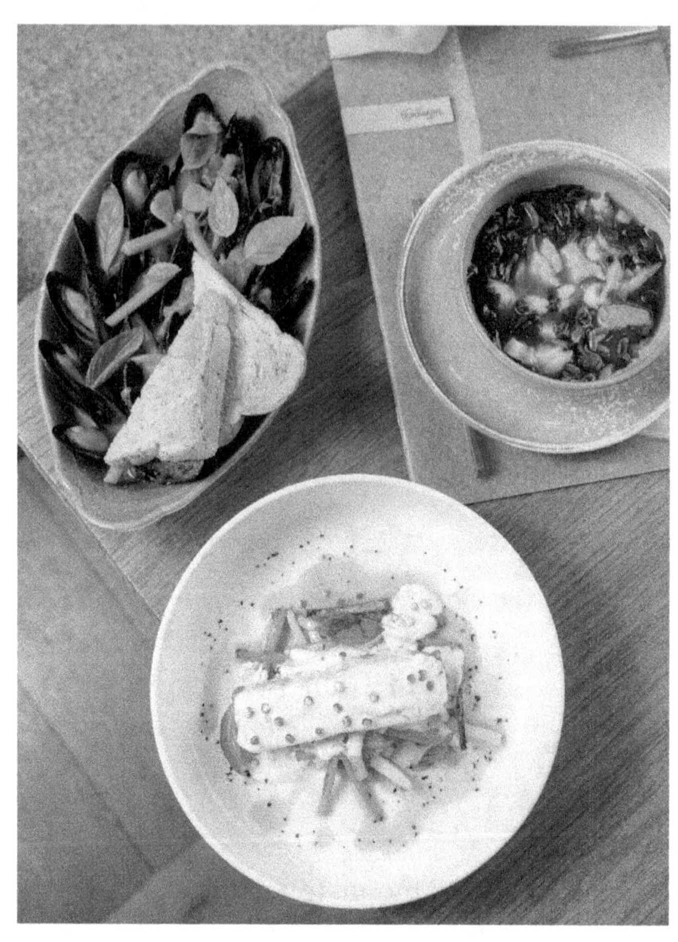

CHAPTER 4

SOUPS AND SALADS

Soups:

1. **Chicken and Vegetable Soup:**
   - A hearty soup with chicken, carrots, celery, and spinach in a flavorful broth.

2. **Tomato Basil Soup:**
   - Ripe tomatoes, fresh basil, garlic, and onions blended into a smooth and comforting soup.

3. **Lentil Soup:**
   - Nutrient-rich lentils cooked with vegetables, spices, and a hint of lemon.

4. **Butternut Squash and Apple Soup:**

- Roasted butternut squash, apples, onions, and warming spices create a sweet and savory soup.

5. **Spicy Thai Shrimp Soup (Tom Yum):**

   - Shrimp, mushrooms, lemongrass, and Thai spices in a tangy and spicy broth.

6. **Quinoa Vegetable Soup:**

   - Quinoa, mixed vegetables, and herbs in a wholesome and protein-packed broth.

7. **Broccoli and Cheddar Soup:**

   - Creamy soup with broccoli florets, cheddar cheese, and a touch of nutmeg.

8. **Chickpea and Spinach Stew:**

- Chickpeas, tomatoes, spinach, and spices simmered into a satisfying stew.

Salads:

1. **Mango Avocado Salad:**
   - Mixed greens with ripe mango, creamy avocado, red onion, and a citrus vinaigrette.
2. **Caesar Salad with Shrimp:**
   - Crisp romaine lettuce, grilled shrimp, croutons, and Caesar dressing.
3. **Cobb Salad:**
   - Grilled chicken, avocado, bacon, hard-boiled eggs, tomatoes, and blue cheese on a bed of mixed greens.
4. **Mediterranean Quinoa Salad:**
   - Quinoa, cherry tomatoes, cucumber, feta cheese, olives, and a lemon-oregano dressing.
5. **Caprese Salad with Balsamic Glaze:**

- ○ Sliced tomatoes, fresh mozzarella, basil, and a drizzle of balsamic glaze.
6. **Spinach Strawberry Salad:**
    - ○ Baby spinach, sliced strawberries, feta cheese, and candied pecans with a balsamic vinaigrette.
7. **Asian Sesame Chicken Salad:**
    - ○ Grilled chicken, mixed greens, mandarin oranges, almonds, and sesame seeds with a sesame-ginger dressing.
8. **Kale and Quinoa Salad with Lemon Tahini Dressing:**
    - ○ Nutrient-packed kale and quinoa with cherry tomatoes, cucumber, and a zesty lemon-tahini dressing.

Feel free to mix and match these recipes or customize them based on your preferences. These soups and salads offer a variety of flavors and textures for a well-rounded and satisfying meal selection.

CHAPTER 5

SANDWICHES AND SPREADS

Sandwiches:

1. **Classic Turkey and Swiss:**
   - Sliced turkey, Swiss cheese, lettuce, and tomato on whole-grain bread.
2. **Caprese Panini:**
   - Fresh mozzarella, tomato, basil, and a drizzle of balsamic glaze on ciabatta bread.
3. **Chicken Avocado Wrap:**
   - Grilled chicken, avocado slices, lettuce, and a light mayo or Greek yogurt dressing wrapped in a whole-grain tortilla.
4. **BLT with Avocado:**
   - Crispy bacon, lettuce, tomato, and sliced avocado on toasted bread.
5. **Vegetarian Hummus Wrap:**
   - Hummus, roasted vegetables (bell peppers, zucchini, eggplant),

spinach, and feta cheese in a
wrap.

6. **Grilled Cheese with Pesto:**
   - Melted cheddar or mozzarella cheese with a spread of basil pesto on sourdough bread.
7. **Tuna Salad Sandwich:**
   - Tuna salad (tuna, mayo, celery, and spices) with lettuce and tomato on whole-grain bread.
8. **Mediterranean Veggie Sandwich:**
   - Hummus, cucumber, red onion, tomato, feta cheese, and olives on multigrain bread.

Spreads:

1. **Basil Pesto:**
   - Fresh basil, garlic, pine nuts, Parmesan cheese, and olive oil blended into a flavorful spread.
2. **Roasted Red Pepper Hummus:**
   - Hummus blended with roasted red peppers for a smoky and savory spread.
3. **Avocado Lime Crema:**

- Creamy avocado mixed with Greek yogurt, lime juice, and a pinch of salt.

4. **Garlic Aioli:**
   - Mayonnaise mixed with minced garlic, lemon juice, and a dash of Dijon mustard.

5. **Chipotle Mayo:**
   - Mayo with chipotle peppers in adobo sauce for a spicy and smoky kick.

6. **Cranberry Walnut Cream Cheese:**
   - Cream cheese blended with dried cranberries and chopped walnuts.

7. **Sun-Dried Tomato Spread:**
   - Sun-dried tomatoes, cream cheese, garlic, and herbs blended into a tangy spread.

8. **Honey Mustard Sauce:**
   - Equal parts honey and Dijon mustard mixed with a touch of lemon juice for a sweet and tangy flavor.

These combinations offer a variety of tastes and textures, making your sandwiches not only delicious but also satisfying. Feel free to mix

and match to create your favorite sandwich
and spread combinations!

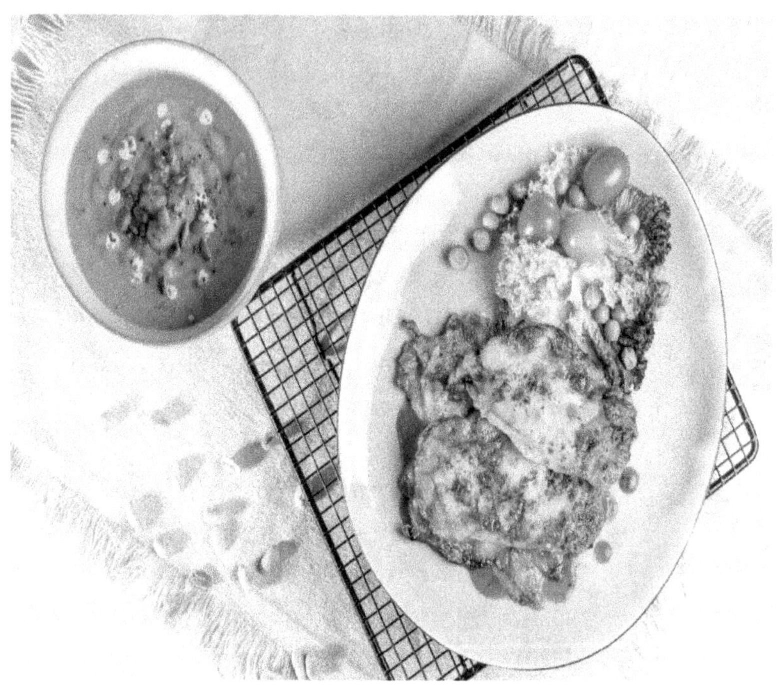

CHAPTER 6

VEGETARIAN AND VEGAN ENTREES

Vegetarian Entrées:

1. **Eggplant Parmesan:**
   - Sliced eggplant coated in breadcrumbs, baked, and layered with marinara sauce and melted mozzarella.
2. **Spinach and Feta Stuffed Portobello Mushrooms:**
   - Portobello mushrooms stuffed with a mixture of spinach, feta cheese, garlic, and breadcrumbs.
3. **Vegetarian Stir-Fry:**
   - Colorful stir-fried vegetables like bell peppers, broccoli, carrots, and tofu in a savory soy-ginger sauce.
4. **Caprese Stuffed Bell Peppers:**
   - Bell peppers filled with a mixture of cherry tomatoes, fresh mozzarella, basil, and balsamic glaze.

5. **Mushroom Risotto:**
   - Creamy risotto made with arborio rice, vegetable broth, white wine, and sautéed mushrooms.
6. **Vegetable Curry:**
   - A medley of vegetables cooked in a flavorful curry sauce served with rice or naan.
7. **Three Cheese Spinach Lasagna:**
   - Layered lasagna with spinach, ricotta, mozzarella, and marinara sauce.
8. **Quinoa-Stuffed Acorn Squash:**
   - Roasted acorn squash halves filled with a mixture of quinoa, black beans, corn, and spices.

Vegan Entrées:

1. **Vegan Chickpea and Vegetable Stir-Fry:**
   - Chickpeas, broccoli, bell peppers, and snap peas stir-fried in a sesame-ginger sauce.
2. **Vegan Lentil Shepherd's Pie:**

o   Lentils cooked with vegetables, topped with mashed sweet potatoes, and baked until golden.

3. **Vegan Eggplant and Chickpea Curry:**
    o   Eggplant and chickpeas simmered in a coconut milk-based curry sauce with aromatic spices.

4. **Vegan Spaghetti Bolognese:**
    o   Lentil or mushroom-based Bolognese sauce served over whole-grain or gluten-free spaghetti.

5. **Stuffed Bell Peppers with Quinoa and Black Beans:**
    o   Bell peppers filled with a mixture of quinoa, black beans, corn, tomatoes, and spices.

6. **Vegan Mushroom and Spinach Wellington:**
    o   Mushrooms and spinach wrapped in puff pastry for a flavorful and festive entrée.

7. **Vegan Buddha Bowl:**
    o   A colorful bowl with a variety of roasted or sautéed vegetables, grains, and a flavorful sauce.

8. **Vegan Chickpea Tikka Masala:**

- Chickpeas cooked in a rich and creamy tomato-based sauce with Indian spices.

These recipes provide a range of textures and flavors, showcasing the versatility of vegetarian and vegan cooking. Whether you're looking for a hearty comfort dish or a light and vibrant option, there's something for every palate.

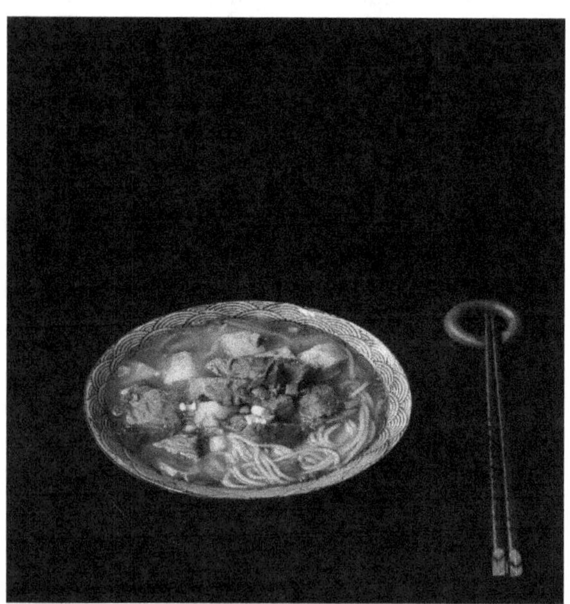

CHAPTER 7

SEAFOOD ENTREES

1. **Grilled Lemon Herb Salmon:**
   - Salmon fillets marinated in a mixture of lemon juice, olive oil, garlic, and fresh herbs, then grilled to perfection.
2. **Shrimp Scampi:**
   - Shrimp cooked in a flavorful sauce made with garlic, white wine, lemon juice, and butter, served over pasta or rice.
3. **Seared Tuna Steaks with Wasabi Mayo:**
   - Ahi tuna steaks seasoned with sesame seeds, seared briefly, and served with a zesty wasabi mayonnaise.
4. **Lemon Garlic Butter Scallops:**
   - Scallops seared in a skillet with a lemon garlic butter sauce, creating a succulent and savory dish.
5. **Cajun Blackened Red Snapper:**

- Red snapper fillets coated in a Cajun spice blend, then pan-seared or grilled for a spicy and flavorful meal.

6. **Lobster Risotto:**
    - Creamy risotto cooked with lobster meat, shallots, white wine, and finished with Parmesan cheese.

7. **Grilled Swordfish with Mango Salsa:**
    - Swordfish steaks seasoned and grilled, topped with a refreshing mango salsa.

8. **Crab-Stuffed Mushrooms:**
    - Mushrooms stuffed with a mixture of crab meat, cream cheese, breadcrumbs, and herbs, then baked until golden.

9. **Baked Lemon Garlic Butter Shrimp:**
    - Shrimp baked in a lemon garlic butter sauce with herbs and served with crusty bread for dipping.

10. **Miso Glazed Cod:**
    - Cod fillets marinated in a miso glaze and then baked or broiled until caramelized and tender.

11. **Coconut Curry Mussels:**

- ○ Fresh mussels cooked in a coconut milk-based curry sauce with aromatics like ginger, garlic, and lemongrass.
12. **Pan-Seared Halibut with Tomato Basil Salsa:**
    - ○ Halibut fillets pan-seared to perfection and topped with a vibrant salsa made with tomatoes, basil, and balsamic vinegar.

These seafood entrées showcase a variety of cooking methods and flavor profiles, allowing you to explore different tastes and textures in your seafood dishes.

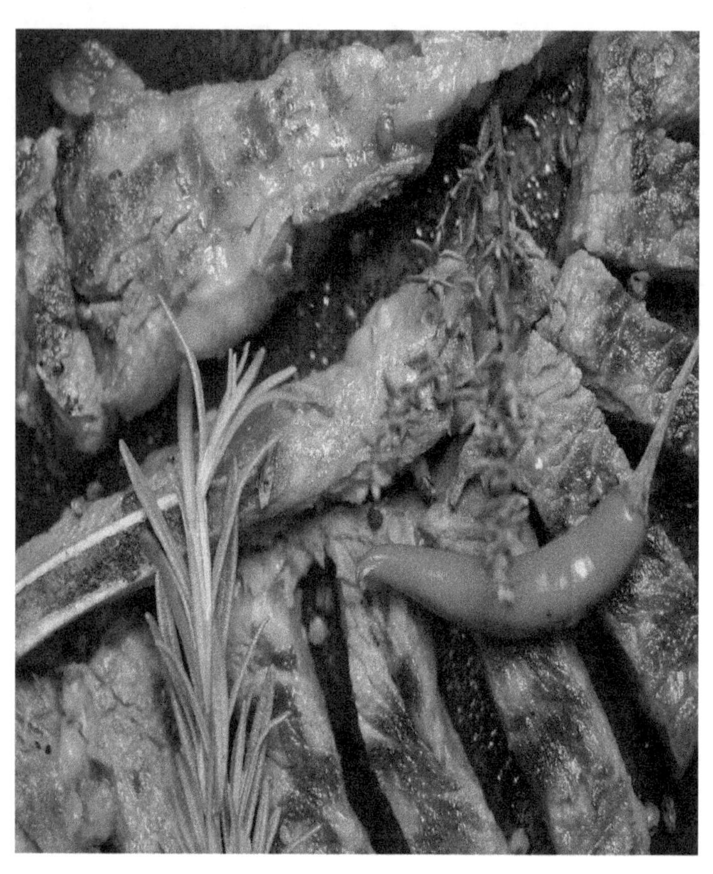

CHAPTER 7

POULTRY AND BEEF ENTRÉES

Poultry Entrée: Balsamic Glazed Chicken with Rosemary

Ingredients:

- 4 boneless, skinless chicken breasts
- Salt and pepper to taste
- 2 tablespoons olive oil
- 1/4 cup balsamic vinegar
- 2 tablespoons honey
- 2 cloves garlic, minced
- 1 teaspoon fresh rosemary, chopped
- 1/2 cup chicken broth
- Fresh rosemary sprigs for garnish

Instructions:

1. Season chicken breasts with salt and pepper.

2. Heat the olive oil in a big skillet over medium-high heat.
3. Add chicken breasts to the skillet and cook for 5-6 minutes per side or until golden brown and cooked through.
4. In a small bowl, whisk together balsamic vinegar, honey, minced garlic, and chopped rosemary.
5. Pour the balsamic mixture over the chicken in the skillet.
6. Add chicken broth to the skillet, stirring to combine. Give it another two to three minutes to simmer.
7. Serve the chicken with the balsamic glaze spooned over the top.
8. Garnish with fresh rosemary sprigs.

Beef Entrée: Beef Tenderloin with Red Wine Reduction

Ingredients:

- 4 beef tenderloin steaks
- Salt and pepper to taste
- 2 tablespoons olive oil
- 1/2 cup red wine
- 1/4 cup beef broth

- 2 tablespoons unsalted butter
- 2 cloves garlic, minced
- 1 teaspoon fresh thyme leaves
- Salt and pepper to taste

Instructions:

1. Preheat the oven to 400°F (200°C).
2. Season beef tenderloin steaks with salt and pepper.
3. In an oven-safe skillet, heat olive oil over high heat.
4. The steaks should be seared for two to three minutes on each side, or until browned.
5. Transfer the skillet to the preheated oven and roast for 10-12 minutes for medium-rare or longer according to your preference.
6. Once the steaks are taken out of the skillet, allow them to rest.
7. In the same skillet over medium heat, add red wine, beef broth, minced garlic, and fresh thyme leaves.
8. Simmer until the sauce is reduced by half. Stir in butter and season with salt and pepper.

9. Serve the beef tenderloin steaks with the red wine reduction sauce drizzled over the top.

Beef Entrée: Beef and Vegetable Stir-Fry

Ingredients:

- 1 pound beef sirloin, thinly sliced
- 2 tablespoons soy sauce
- 1 tablespoon oyster sauce
- 1 tablespoon hoisin sauce
- 1 tablespoon cornstarch
- 2 tablespoons vegetable oil, divided
- 2 bell peppers, sliced
- 1 broccoli crown, cut into florets
- 1 carrot, julienned
- 3 cloves garlic, minced
- 1 tablespoon fresh ginger, grated
- Green onions for garnish
- Cooked rice for serving

Instructions:

1. In a bowl, combine soy sauce, oyster sauce, hoisin sauce, and cornstarch to create a marinade.
2. Place sliced beef in the marinade and let it marinate for at least 20 minutes.
3. In a big skillet or wok, heat up one tablespoon of vegetable oil on high heat.
4. Stir-fry the marinated beef until browned. Take out of the wok and place aside.
5. Add another tablespoon of oil to the same wok.
6. Stir-fry garlic and ginger until fragrant.
7. Add sliced bell peppers, broccoli, and julienned carrots to the wok. Stir-fry for 3-4 minutes until vegetables are crisp-tender.
8. Return the cooked beef to the wok and toss everything together until well combined and heated through.
9. Garnish with green onions and serve over cooked rice.

Poultry Entrée: Baked Lemon Garlic Chicken Breast

Ingredients:

- 4 boneless, skinless chicken breasts
- 4 tablespoons olive oil
- 4 cloves garlic, minced
- Juice of 2 lemons
- Zest of 1 lemon
- 1 teaspoon dried thyme
- Salt and pepper to taste
- Fresh parsley for garnish

Instructions:

1. Preheat the oven to 400°F (200°C).
2. Place chicken breasts in a baking dish.
3. In a bowl, whisk together olive oil, minced garlic, lemon juice, lemon zest, dried thyme, salt, and pepper.
4. Thoroughly coat the chicken breasts with the marinade by pouring it over them.
5. Bake in the preheated oven for 25-30 minutes or until the chicken reaches an internal temperature of 165°F (74°C).
6. Optional: Broil for an additional 2-3 minutes for a golden finish.
7. Garnish with fresh parsley and serve.

Beef Entrée: Beef and Mushroom Stroganoff

Ingredients:

- 1 pound beef sirloin or tenderloin, thinly sliced
- 2 tablespoons olive oil
- 1 onion, finely chopped
- 2 cups mushrooms, sliced
- 3 cloves garlic, minced
- 2 tablespoons all-purpose flour
- 1 cup beef broth
- 1 tablespoon Worcestershire sauce
- 1 tablespoon Dijon mustard
- 1/2 cup sour cream
- Salt and pepper to taste
- Fresh parsley for garnish
- Cooked egg noodles or rice for serving

Instructions:

1. Heat the olive oil in a big skillet over medium-high heat.
2. Add sliced beef and cook until browned. After taking the steak out of the skillet, set it aside.

3. In the same skillet, add chopped onion and sliced mushrooms. Sauté until softened.
4. Add the minced garlic and continue cooking for one more minute.
5. After dusting the vegetables with flour, mix them together.
6. Gradually pour in beef broth, Worcestershire sauce, and Dijon mustard. Stir until the mixture thickens.
7. Return the cooked beef to the skillet and simmer for 5-7 minutes.
8. Stir in sour cream and season with salt and pepper.
9. Serve rice or cooked egg noodles with the beef and mushroom stroganoff.
10. Garnish with fresh parsley before serving.

Poultry Entrée: Lemon Rosemary Roast Chicken

Ingredients:

- 4 bone-in, skin-on chicken thighs
- 2 tablespoons olive oil
- 2 tablespoons fresh rosemary, chopped

- Zest of 1 lemon
- Juice of 1 lemon
- 4 cloves garlic, minced
- Salt and pepper to taste
- Lemon slices for garnish

Instructions:

1. Preheat the oven to 400°F (200°C).
2. In a small bowl, mix together olive oil, chopped rosemary, lemon zest, lemon juice, minced garlic, salt, and pepper.
3. Place chicken thighs in a roasting pan or baking dish.
4. Brush the chicken thighs with the lemon rosemary mixture, ensuring they are well coated.
5. Roast in the preheated oven for 35-40 minutes or until the chicken reaches an internal temperature of 165°F (74°C) and the skin is golden brown.
6. Garnish with lemon slices before serving.

These poultry and beef entrées are sure to impress with their rich flavors and elegant presentations. Enjoy your delicious meals!

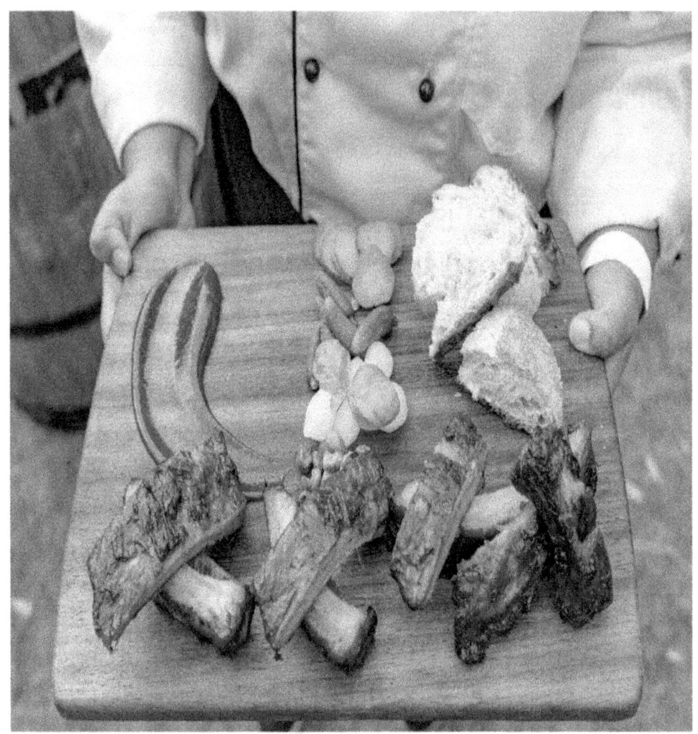

CHAPTER 7

SWEET TREATS

Classic Chocolate Brownies:

Ingredients:

- 1 cup (2 sticks) unsalted butter
- 2 cups granulated sugar
- 4 large eggs
- 1 teaspoon vanilla extract
- 1 cup all-purpose flour
- 1/2 cup cocoa powder
- 1/4 teaspoon baking powder
- 1/4 teaspoon salt
- 1 cup chocolate chips (optional)

Instructions:

1. Preheat the oven to 350°F (175°C) and grease a 9x13-inch baking pan.

2. Melt the butter in a saucepan over low
    heat. Remove from heat and stir in
    sugar, eggs, and vanilla extract.
3. In a separate bowl, whisk together flour,
    cocoa powder, baking powder, and salt.
4. Mixing just until combined, add the dry
    ingredients to the wet ones. If desired,
    fold in chocolate chips.
5. Evenly distribute the batter after pouring
    it into the baking pan.
6. Bake for 25 to 30 minutes, or until moist
    crumbs come out of a toothpick inserted
    in the center.
7. Before slicing the brownies into squares,
    let them cool.

Fresh Strawberry Shortcake:

Ingredients:

- 1 pound fresh strawberries, hulled and
  sliced
- 1/4 cup granulated sugar
- 2 cups all-purpose flour
- 1/4 cup granulated sugar (for the
  shortcakes)
- 1 tablespoon baking powder

- 1/2 teaspoon salt
- 1/2 cup unsalted butter, cold and cubed
- 3/4 cup milk
- 1 teaspoon vanilla extract
- Whipped cream for topping

Instructions:

1. In a bowl, combine sliced strawberries with 1/4 cup sugar. Give them about thirty minutes to macerate.
2. Adjust the oven temperature to 425°F (220°C) and place parchment paper on a baking sheet.
3. Mix the flour, baking powder, 1/4 cup sugar, and salt in a big bowl.
4. Add the cubed, cold butter and cut until the mixture is the consistency of coarse crumbs.
5. Add milk and vanilla extract, stirring until well combined.
6. Drop spoonfuls of the dough onto the prepared baking sheet to form shortcakes.
7. Bake until golden brown, 12 to 15 minutes.

8. Allow the shortcakes to cool, then slice them in half horizontally.

9. Spoon macerated strawberries onto the bottom half of each shortcake, add a dollop of whipped cream, and place the top half over the filling.

Chocolate Chip Cookies:

Ingredients:

- 1 cup (2 sticks) unsalted butter, softened
- 3/4 cup granulated sugar
- 3/4 cup packed brown sugar
- 2 large eggs
- 1 teaspoon vanilla extract
- 2 1/4 cups all-purpose flour
- 1 teaspoon baking soda
- 1/2 teaspoon salt
- 2 cups chocolate chips
- 1 cup chopped nuts (optional)

Instructions:

1. Preheat the oven to 375°F (190°C).

2. In a large bowl, beat together softened butter, granulated sugar, brown sugar, eggs, and vanilla extract until creamy.
3. Mix the baking soda, salt, and flour in a different bowl. Mix thoroughly after adding the dry ingredients to the wet ones gradually.
4. Stir in chocolate chips and nuts (if using).
5. Drop dough onto ungreased baking sheets in rounded tablespoons.
6. Bake in the preheated oven for 9-11 minutes or until golden brown.
7. After a few minutes, let the cookies cool on the baking sheets before moving them to wire racks to finish cooling.

Fresh Fruit Parfait:

Ingredients:

- 2 cups Greek yogurt
- 2 tablespoons honey
- 1 teaspoon vanilla extract
- 1 cup granola

- 2 cups mixed fresh fruits (berries, kiwi, mango, etc.)
- Mint leaves for garnish (optional)

Instructions:

1. In a bowl, mix Greek yogurt, honey, and vanilla extract until well combined.
2. In serving glasses or bowls, layer the bottom with a spoonful of the yogurt mixture.
3. Add a layer of granola over the yogurt.
4. Top with a layer of mixed fresh fruits.
5. Repeat the layers until the glasses are filled, finishing with a layer of fresh fruits on top.
6. Garnish with mint leaves if desired.
7. Serve immediately and enjoy!

CONCLUSION

In conclusion, exploring a variety of heart-healthy recipes, understanding the importance of preventive measures against heart disease, and incorporating a balanced Mediterranean diet can contribute significantly to overall well-being.

- Heart Health at the Center: The Mediterranean diet takes center stage as a key player in promoting a healthy heart.
- Nutrient-Rich and Balanced: Emphasizing nutrient-rich, balanced meals, the Mediterranean diet provides a wealth of fruits, vegetables, whole grains, and lean proteins.
- Diverse and Delicious Choices: Exploring heart-healthy recipes, such as Quinoa-Stuffed Bell Peppers and Chocolate Chip Cookies, adds variety to meals while supporting cardiovascular health.
- Mindful Nutrition: Understanding the heart truth, recognizing common risks, and being aware of types of heart

disease empower individuals to make informed choices for heart health.

- Holistic Approach: Beyond the plate, incorporating regular physical activity, stress management, and maintaining a healthy weight are crucial factors in achieving and maintaining cardiovascular wellness.
- Every Meal Matters: Whether enjoying a nourishing breakfast, crafting satisfying sandwiches, or indulging in sweet treats, each meal presents an opportunity to contribute to heart disease prevention.
- Importance of Eating Healthy for the Heart:
    - Reduces the risk of heart disease and related complications.
    - Helps maintain healthy cholesterol levels.
    - Supports overall cardiovascular well-being.
    - Contributes to weight management and optimal blood pressure.

In essence, making conscious and nutritious choices in our daily meals is a proactive step

towards a heart-healthy lifestyle, contributing to
our overall health and well-being.

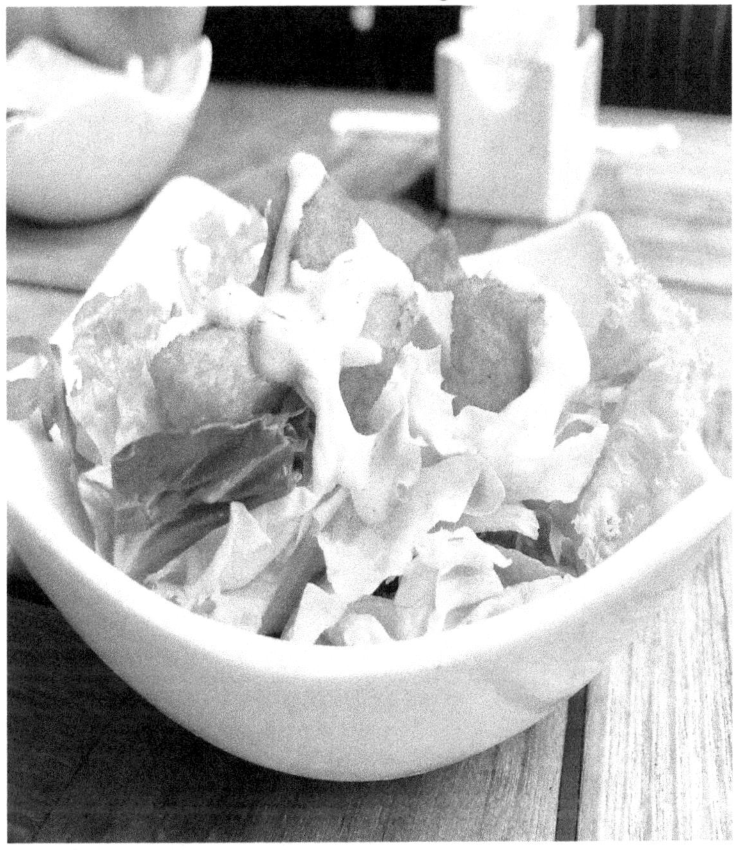

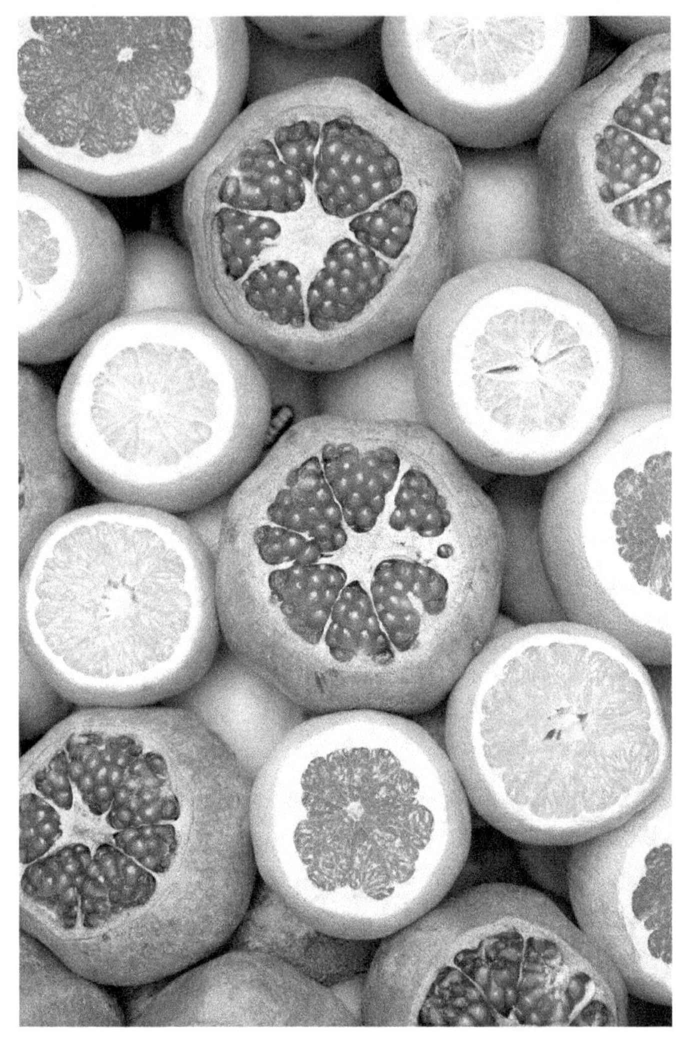